PREPARING FOR A LOCKDOWN

A FAMILY GUIDE TO STAYING SAFE.

SILVERGUM PUBLISHING

| SILVERGUM PUBLISHING

ISBN-13: 9780648390879
ISBN-10: 0648390879

Cover design by: Silvergum Publishing
Layout Book Design Templates

Disclaimer

The information provided in this book is of a general nature and to be used as a guide only. Any medical conditions should be seen to by a medical practitioner.

Australian spelling and metric measures are used throughout the book.

Contents

What you will need for a short-term lockdown. 1

Top Tips 3

Food Supplies 5

Medical Supplies 19

Sanitary Supplies 23

Pets 25

Entertainment 27

Backyard Self Sufficiency 29

Make a Plan of Action 33

Prepare your home for a lockdown 35

Preventing Infection 37

10 tips to make life in isolation easier 39

Back up your electronics 41

Stock up on Batteries 43

Assess your lighting needs 47

How much water do you need? 51

How to freeze vegetables 53

How to sanitize your food 59

Learn to cook in a crisis 61

Before and during a storm 65

After a Disaster 67

Easy Recipes for a lockdown 69

   Chicken and vegetable Ramen noodles 69

   Beef and Bean Enchiladas or Bean Enchiladas 71

   One pot cauliflower, chicken and rice 75

Creamy chicken fettuccine 77

Creamy tuna pasta bake 79

Chicken with Cashew nuts 81

Chilli con carne 83

Curry cauliflower soup 85

Baked Spaghetti 87

Chicken or Salmon Yakitori Skewers 89

Shepard's Pie Parcels 91

Vegetarian Bolognese 93

One pot lemon chicken and rice 95

Mexican beef and rice casserole 97

Apple Pikelets /flapjacks 99

Flour Tortillas 101

Making bread by hand 103

Make your own hand sanitizer 105

Make an Oral Rehydration preparation 107

Acknowledgments 109

Introduction

There are many books on preparing or *prepping* for a long-term worldwide disaster such as an EMP blast, nuclear war or meteor strike. ***Preparing for a Lockdown*** focuses on what you need to do in a short-term crisis to keep your family safe and fed. This includes an event such as a power outage, pandemic, flood, cyclone, hurricane or any other event that forces your family into a lockdown or self-isolation.

In 2017 Hurricane Katrina caused widespread damage and loss throughout New Orleans in 2019 Typhoon Odai killed over 900 people in Africa, and in early 2020 bushfires ravaged Australia and an unexpected pandemic hit the world. Movie theatres, gyms, schools, restaurants and many other services we take for granted were shut down. Many countries saw panic buying of goods such as hand sanitizer, toilet paper, rice, pasta and medical supplies. Shelves were left bare and restrictions were placed on purchases. Families were forced to quarantine inside their homes, international travel was placed on hold and countries were placed in lockdown as Governments tried to stem the spread of infection.

Many people were unprepared for these disasters and unsure what they needed to keep their families safe.

Preparing for a Lockdown will provide you with a guideline of what you will need if your family is placed in a short-term lockdown or self-isolation due to a power outage, natural disaster or pandemic. You can also extend this period with added supplies.

Easy recipes are included at the back of the book, using food and items from your pantry.

Stay safe and remember to *hope for the best, prepare for the worst!*

What you will need for a short-term lockdown.

If your family must go into quarantine, or you want to be prepared in case of a lockdown, power failure or natural disaster, here are useful tips on what you will need without going on a wild spending spree. Some of the foods and items you will already have in your home. The foods and items can be adjusted to suit your own family's tastes and size.

TIPS Purchase what your family likes to eat, and you feel comfortable preparing. If you purchase twenty tins of tomatoes just because everyone else is, however, you hate tomatoes they will only take up space in your home and be a waste of your money.

Be prepared to substitute. You may not have the exact ingredients for a particular meal you want to make, and you won't be able to *pop to the shops* to buy it. Instead substitute. For example, substitute rice instead of pasta or spaghetti, use different beans, vegetables, herbs and spices. Don't be afraid to get creative.

Freeze leftovers

Freeze chopped fruit and vegetables for use in cooking (see below for tips of which vegetable and fruits freeze well).

Freeze plastic bags or containers of water. These can be used in a cooler/esky to help keep food cold, or for drinking water once thawed.

Have alternate cooking methods available to use in case of power outages (see chapter on cooking in a disaster.)

Top Tips

- **Shop at the right times** find out when stores do major restocking. Opening times are ideal e.g. 7 am.

- **Skip bread.** Buy tortillas/wraps instead. These are compact and versatile and can be stored in your pantry.

- **Buy stock cubes and powder** instead of stock in cartons as it is cheaper and more space efficient.

- **Know what can be frozen** Read the list below.

- **Buy your essential herbs and spices** See list below.

- **Buy your essential sauces** See list below.

  If you have a good supply of stock, herbs spices and sauces you can make anything taste delicious!

- **Tinned Tomatoes** Can't find tinned tomatoes? You can make a substitute by mixing 1 ½ Tablespoons flour with 1/4 cup of water and whisk together until lump free. Add another 1 ¼ cups of water, plus 4 Tablespoons of tomato paste and 1 Teaspoon of sugar. Bring to simmer on stove until mixture thickens to your liking. This can be used in place of 1 can of tomatoes.

- **Skip fast food/uber eats** particularly from chain restaurants where a lot of people might be visiting.

Food Supplies

<u>Tinned Food</u>

Tinned vegetables e.g. corn, peas, beans, carrots.

Tinned soup

Tinned ready meals

Tinned fish e.g. tuna, salmon, sardines

Tinned fruits

Baby food

Tinned beans and legumes

Tinned spaghetti/pasta

Dried Packaged Foods

Cereals e.g. porridge/oats

Pasta (spaghetti, noodles, instant, egg noodles and rice noodles)

Rice

Instant Noodles

Dried pasta meals

Powdered milk and baby formula

Flour

Corn flour

Baking powder/bi-carb soda

Sugar (brown and white)

Yeast

Bread mix

Tea/coffee/hot chocolate/Milo

Nuts (e.g. cashews, almonds, peanuts both salted and unsalted)

Pancake mix

Tomato paste (this can be used as a substitute for tinned tomatoes – see recipe under the top tips)

Corn chips

Packet cake and muffin mixes

Peanut butter/honey/vegemite/hazelnut spread/jam etc.

Herbs and spices

Salt and pepper

Onion

Garlic

Cumin

Coriander

Paprika

Oregano

Thyme

Chilli powder or Cayenne pepper

Curry powder

Mustard powder

Beef, vegetable and chicken stock powder or stock cubes (1 cube or 1 tsp powder in 1 cup / 250 ml boiling water = 1 cup stock).

Sauces

Tomato

BBQ

Worcestershire

Soy

Oyster

Sweet chilli

Gravy

Mirin

Chinese cooking wine

Sesame oil

Red wine vinegar

Perishables

TIP Make sure you check the use by dates on your perishables and freeze or use them before the expiry date as they may not last the full two weeks of the lockdown.

Beef, lamb, pork, chicken and fish or vegan alternatives. (These can also be frozen to extend their use-by date).

Milk/soymilk/almond milk etc. (long life and powdered versions of these can be purchased)

Cheeses- parmesan, tasty, mozzarella etc. (grated parmesan and mozzarella/tasty chesses can be frozen)

Cream/sour cream (these can be frozen)
Fruit and vegetables (cut into small chunks and freeze in zip lock bags)

Eggs (these will keep in the fridge for several months)

Juice (box juices last longer)

Yogurt

Cold meats e.g. ham, bacon, salami (these can be frozen in bits)

Butter (can also be frozen in cubes)

Vegetables

Buy a variety of vegetables from tinned, fresh and frozen. You can also freeze your own using zip lock bags, these can then be used in cooking.

Vegetables that can be frozen:

capsicum/bell peppers

onions brown, white and red

garlic

ginger

carrot

celery

corn

pumpkin

squash

zucchini

cauliflower

broccoli / broccolini

spinach

kale

limes (remove skin first and cut into wedges)

lemons (remove skin first and cut into wedges)

spring onions

(See section at the rear of the book on how to freeze vegetables).

<u>**Vegetable that have a long shelf life:**</u>

Potatoes

Cabbage

Carrots

Sweet potato

Brussel sprouts

Beetroot

Parsnip

Cauliflower

Onions

Spring onions

Garlic

Ginger

Vegetables such as lettuce, baby spinach, cucumbers tomatoes and other leafy greens have a shorter shelf life and don't freeze well. Do not purchase too many of these.

Fruit

Extend the life of your fruit by keeping it in the fridge especially in hot weather.

Freeze chopped fruit in zip lock bags for use in smoothies, slushies and cakes.

Fruit that freezes well includes
Berries (blueberries, raspberries, strawberries)

Bananas (skin removed)

Mango

Pineapple

Apples

Tinned fruit and dried fruit are also a good alternative to fresh fruit and can be used in cooking.

Freezer

Beef, lamb, pork, chicken and fish

Vegetables

Fruit packs

Pizza or other ready meals

Bread/Rolls

Ready rolled pastry

Fresh vegetables such as capsicum/bell peppers, and onions can be chopped and frozen in zip lock bags for later use.

Fresh peeled bananas, blueberries, mango and raspberries can be frozen in zip lock bags for later use.

Egg white can be frozen and used in cooking

Water and liquids

Bottled water. It is wise to have a small supply of bottled water available, however, tap water is fine to drink.

Bottled juice.

Long life milk, Almond milk/soy milk etc.

Coconut water/juice/milk

Stock e.g. beef, chicken, vegetable. (Stock cubes can also be used)

Some soft drinks

Alcohol

Cooking oil, olive, vegetable, coconut, peanut

Treats

TIP It's not much fun having to go into lockdown, especially with kids, so a few treats your family enjoys eating is a good idea. Just don't go overboard as you will probably be doing a lot of sitting around and not a lot of exercising! Loading your body with sugar will not help your immune system either.

Examples of treats include chocolate, ice cream, chips, popcorn, cakes and biscuits. You can also make your own if you prefer a healthier option.

Medical Supplies

TIP Make sure you have enough supply of your usual prescription medicines to last at least a month. Even if you are only going into lockdown for two weeks, it may take time for pharmacies to restock their supplies.

Thermometer

Contraceptive pill/condoms

Contact lenses and solution

Spare glasses

Pain relief/Paracetamol/ children's paracetamol

Cough suppressant

Nasal decongestant

Oral rehydration sachets (or make your own - see recipe at back of this book)

heartburn relief

constipation relief

anti-nausea and anti-diarrhea

anti-biotic cream

antifungal cream

antihistamine cream and tablets

isopropyl alcohol and/or peroxide

sharp scissors

Lozenges for sore throat.

Band-aids (plasters)

Antiseptic cream

Antiseptic cleaner

TIP as your access to fresh fruit and vegetables, and time outside in the sunshine may be limited, some vitamins may be beneficial. Read the packet instructions for how much to consume. More is not always better.

Some examples include:

Multi-vitamins and minerals

Vitamin C 1000mg

Vitamin D

Zinc

Calcium

Sanitary Supplies

Hand sanitizer (if it is available!)

Soap/body wash/hand wash

Deodorant

Toothpaste

Mouth wash (containing alcohol for killing germs)

Tampons/pads

Shampoo and conditioner

Chapstick

Body lotion

Tissues

Toilet paper (2-3 rolls per person per week)

Baby nappies/diapers and related products (wipes, creams etc.)

Other household products

Paper towels (these can be used for drying hands rather than hand towels)

Clothes detergent

Cleaning products

Bleach/disinfectant

Dishwashing liquid/dishwasher tablets and powder

Aluminum foil and cling wrap, baking paper

Garbage bags

Matches

Candles

Torch

Batteries

Zip lock bags (good for freezing cut up fruit and vegetables)

Steel wool (you can start a fire for a wood burner if you don't have matches by rubbing the steel wool against a 9-volt battery.)

Pets

Don't forget your pets! Make sure you have enough pet food available for at least three weeks. Visit your vet to ensure their immunizations are up to date.

Pet food tinned and dried for dogs and cats.

Litter tray and litter refills

Fish food

Seed for birds

Hay and pellets for rabbits, guinea pigs, mice, chickens etc.

Maybe a new toy to keep them occupied if you are not able to take them outside for a few days

Entertainment

Okay, so going into lockdown is a great time to catch up on Netflix and other tv show/ movies you've been wanting to watch, but you can't sit and watch TV all day (well you can, but, eventually you will get a headache!) Here's some entertainment ideas besides the television and computer to keep your family occupied during lockdown.

Playing Cards

Board games (there are some fun ones out there that cater to lovers of television series such as *Game of Thrones Monopoly and Harry Potter Cluedo*), there's also chess, checkers and other old-style games you may have always wanted to learn.

Yo-Yos (get the kids to take these outside or on the balcony if you don't have a backyard)

Rubik's cube and other puzzle games

Jigsaws

Music

Books! Grab a few books or a series from your local bookstore.

Magazines

Books on tape

A couple of new toys for the kids will keep them occupied for a few days.

Active games such as skipping ropes and basketball that can be played with in your backyard.

Coloured pencils/markers and colouring books or blank books for drawing.

Arts and crafts for the kids or yourself (maybe you've always wanted to try knitting, quilting, dressmaking or woodworking).

Hand weights/ yoga mats/ stretching bands to do some light exercise if you feel you want to burn some energy.

Backyard Self Sufficiency

If you want to take things a step further to being self-sufficient for your lockdown and into the future some ideas, you may want to consider include:

Growing your own vegetable garden. For this you will need a spot with good soil or potting mix with 6 hours of sunlight a day, fertilizer and plenty or water. Easy to grow plants include, lemons, tomatoes, capsicums, potatoes, lettuce and beans.

Grow an indoor garden. For those households without a backyard or limited space, a small window garden, table that sits in the sunshine or balcony can be used. Obviously, you won't be able to grow vegetables that need a lot of space such as potatoes, however, plants such as herbs (parsley, basil, mint, oregano etc.), peppers, cherry tomatoes, and lettuce grow well in pots.

Make sure they are well drained and have adequate sunshine. Growing a garden like this can be great fun for the kids too!

<u>Water tank.</u> For a water tank to work properly it will need a roof to attach to for rainwater runoff. The water can then be used to water your garden or drink if sanitized first.

<u>Solar Power </u>Solar power panels can be added to your house to supplement your electricity supply and you may even be able to sell some back to

your electrical supplier. There are many solar power companies available now offering deals on adding solar power to your house, however, these vary in quality so do your research before purchasing.

<u>Chicken Coop </u> A great way to have a fresh supply of eggs is to keep chickens in your back yard. They will need enough space to roam and a covered nesting area to sleep. You will also need to provide them with hay for bedding, pellets and vegetable scraps for food, plus drinking water. Not all councils and areas allow chickens especially in city areas, so you will need to check your local rules and guidelines before purchasing any poultry. For example, roosters are usually not allowed in suburban areas.

Make your own composter

You can build an outdoor composter using a 110 litre /30-gallon barrel. First drill some holes in the bottom for drainage, then layer 6 inches/ 100 cm of small sticks in the bottom for air circulation. Next layer grass cuttings and kitchen waste (vegetable and fruit scraps, eggshells, tea and coffee grounds. No meat or dairy products.)
Keep the contents moist and roll the barrel around every few days to keep it aerated.
Once the barrel is full it will take approximately 6 weeks to decompose into rich soil for your garden. If you have two compost barrels working you can alternate between them.

Learn First Aid

Every adult in your household and even older children should have some basic first aid training including how to administer CRP (cardiopulmonary resuscitation). First Aid courses are available through the red cross and St Johns Ambulance offices.

Make a Plan of Action

To help your family stay safe, you should have a *family plan of action*. Everyone in the household needs to be aware of this action plan. You can also include other family members (for example, grandparents) and friends if you wish.

For example, an action plan could include:

Make a list of medical and emergency numbers
Keep this list in an easily accessible location for all family members to access if needed. For example, on the refrigerator or a pin-up board.

Who is most at risk in your family?
For example, older people, pregnant women and people with underlying health risks such as asthma or diabetes or compromised immune systems may be more at risk. Speak to your General Practitioner about what extra assistance they might need and how you can minimize any infection. For example, during a pandemic, those at a higher risk may need to eat separately from the family and maintain a distance of 2 meters from other household members.

Where can you isolate if a family member becomes infected

Identify a room/s you can use to isolate one or more of your family members if they become sick/infected. This area will need to be cleaned regularly to help stop the spread of infection to other family members. If you have more than one

bathroom or toilet in your home, dedicate one of the bathrooms/toilets to the sick members of the family.

Prepare your home for a lockdown

Cleaning and sanitizing

Get into the habit of washing your hands regularly with soap and water for 20-minutes, especially when you have been out of the house (for example, at work or buying food/ petrol etc. or at the park with your children).

Regularly clean door handles and cupboard knobs, refrigerator handles, oven and microwave doors, computer keyboard and mouse, and television remote controls. These items would be regularly touched by household members.

For family members working away from the home before a lockdown is enforced, (for example, health care workers and grocery store attendants) have a designated area where they can remove shoes and coats when returning home. Spray these with a disinfectant. These family members should also wash their hands thoroughly or use hand sanitizer before coming into contact with other family members.

Purchase enough food and medical supplies for at least three weeks of isolation. (see previous chapters for ideas and tips on what you may need).

Go Local

Plan to use smaller, local supermarkets, ATMs, petrol/gas stations and pharmacies as they will have less people using them as opposed to the larger centres. Make sure you wash your hands thoroughly or use hand sanitizer after using petrol/gas pumps, ATMS, cash machines, touch screens, elevator buttons, shopping trolly handles or escalator handrails.

Limit the number of visitors coming to your home.

Keep the number of people coming into your home who are not your immediate family to a minimum. The fewer number of people you encounter the risk of becoming infected decreases. Many people will not show outward signs of infection until many days or even weeks after they are contagious.

Sanitize any deliveries

Before bringing any deliveries including letters and parcels into your home, they should be sanitized or left for three hours before handling. Wipe or spray with disinfectant or use gloves and wash your hands with soap and water afterwards.

Preventing Infection

Once a virus has started to spread throughout the community and become a pandemic, the chances of infection increase.
To decrease your risk of infection the Centre of Disease Control recommends:

Keep your distance.
Stay 1.5 to 2 metres away from other people and try to keep away from crowed areas unless absolutely necessary.

Sanitize your hands
Use soap and water to lather and wash your hands for at least 20 minutes, especially if you have been outside your home or in contact with other people. Alcohol based hand sanitizer can also be used.

Stay Hydrated
Drink plenty of warm fluids to keep your body hydrated and to help flush any contaminants from

your throat into your stomach where your stomach acids can help neutralize them.

Sneeze and cough into a tissue.
Try and keep germs away from other people by sneezing or coughing into a tissue and throwing the tissue away. Alternatively sneeze or cough into the crook of your arm. If you cough/sneeze into your hands and then touch something, germs are spread.

Wear a face mask
If you are infected or suspect you are infected, wear a face mask to prevent the spread of germs to other people, particularly members of your household as they will be in close contact with you.

Seek Medical advice
If you are ill or have reason to believe you are infected, seek medical advice and be prepared to self-isolate.

Washing
Wash clothes, shower and wash hair regularly especially after leaving your home to go the supermarket or other areas where many people have been.
https://www.cdc.gov

10 tips to make life in isolation easier

Suddenly having to live in isolation when you are used to being able to go out and do whatever you want, whenever you want can be a challenge Follow these 10 tips to make the experience easier.

Focus on the positives. You're in the comfort of your own home. You get to spend quality time with your family. You can do many of the things you never usually have time for!

Schedule a much-needed job to do each day.

Have a family board game night.

Open your windows each day and let the fresh air in.

Spend some time outside each day even it is only on your balcony or front porch. Vitamin D is good for your health and immunity.

Stay in touch with your relatives and friends by Skype, Messenger, Facetime etc. Being able to see other people is a boost to your mental health.

Keep a diary of your thoughts and what you did during the day. You might find it interesting to look back on your experience in years to come.

Don't spend all your time on the computer or watching TV. Be productive. Do things you've been wanting to do.

Do some exercise even if it's only stretching or walking around your apartment or backyard. There are also plenty of exercise programs on YouTube.

Don't be afraid to tell your family/friends/house-mates that you need some space for a couple of hours. It's not easy to *live on top* of each other and having time to yourself is important. If you find yourself getting frustrated or angry at your situation or your housemates, take a break and do something by yourself.

Back up your electronics

As most of us live our lives on our computers and mobile phones. Our precious videos and photographs of friends and family, work and personal information, contact lists and financial information are all stored on them. Nobody wants to lose this data because of a lightning strike during an electrical storm so you should always prepare your home electronics for any power disruptions and storms.

- Always back up your important data to a thumb drive, the cloud or a portable hard drive.

- Have a NID (network interface device) attached to your home to protect your home's wiring from lightning strikes by directing surges greater than 300 volts into the ground.

- Install a surge protector to protect electronics against voltage spikes and surges.

- An extra level of protection is a UPS (uninterrupted power supply) which will prevent a temporary power disruption to your computer which could cause you to lose valuable data. When there is an abrupt cutting of power to your computer.

- Keep an eye on the weather and if a storm is likely, unplug your computers. It is not enough to switch off at the wall, you must unplug from the power outlet or phone jack.

Stock up on Batteries

You never know when there is going to be a power outage, so it is a good idea to have a supply of spare batteries for torches, radios, lanterns and other devices.

Batteries should be stored at room temperature (putting them in the freezer does not extend their life) and kept in their original packaging. Don't leave any loose batteries jumbled in a box as it's a fire hazard to have them touching each other.

Any batteries that are leaking should be discarded. Don't mix old and new batteries.

Have a range of fully charged batteries including A, AA, AAA, C and D.

There are many different types of batteries including:

Nickel-Cadmium rechargeable (NiCad). These rechargeable batteries have a long shelf life, charge quickly and can be recharged over and over hundreds of times. The do however lose power quickly, even when not in use

Nickel-metal hydride (NiMH). These batteries hold their power longer when not is use so are useful to have as spares.

Alkaline, disposable. These batteries are commonly sold in supermarkets and hardware stores, they are not rechargeable so you will need to keep a supply of them.

Alkaline, rechargeable. These types of battery are rechargeable; however, they need to be disposed of at a recycling facility.

Button style batteries. These batteries are in a lot of devices; however, they are not rechargeable so you will need to keep a supply of them. Because of their small size these batteries are easily swallowed so be sure to keep them out of reach of young children.

Battery Chargers
There a lot of different battery chargers available and you will need to choose one that matches the size battery you want to charge (many are not interchangeable). Some *smart* chargers can read the battery and stop charging once the battery is full, others have a light that changes colour and you will need to turn them off yourself once charging is finished.

Some battery chargers will work off your mains power, some from your car's 12-volt power outlet and some from a solar battery.

Battery Testers

A battery tester is a good investment if your use batteries regularly or you keep your batteries all mixed together in a box. It is a simple gadget that allows you to test your batteries to see whether they still have charge. This can be very useful and takes the frustration out of taking batteries in and out of a torch trying to find ones that work!

Assess your lighting needs

When preparing for a lockdown it is important to assess your lighting needs. In case of a power outage you need to ensure you have adequate lighting for you and your family. This is particularly important if you have small children in the home as blackouts can be frightening.

Torches/flashlights/lanterns

Make sure you have at least one working torch/flashlight in your home that is in easy reach if you are suddenly plunged into darkness. It is preferable to have a medium sized torch/flashlight for each member of the family including children as this will make them feel more secure. Keep these within an easy to reach areas such as the bedrooms, kitchen or laundry (this will depend on the layout of your home).

If you have a double story home or home with an attic or basement, place a torch in these areas too. Navigating stairs in the darkness is can be dangerous.

Check your torches/flashlights regularly to ensure they work, and the batteries and bulbs are functioning. Have spare batteries available in case they need to be changed (see the chapter *Stock up on Batteries*).

Have at least one large light as his is better for illuminating your yard, and assessing dangers such as dangling electrical wires, fallen trees, rising water and suspicious noises).

Some torches have added lens filters such as blue filters which are good for reading maps in the darkness.

Solar Lights

Solar lamps can be very useful; however, they need to be full charged in bright light (the sun) to give off enough light. During a power outage or storm, you won't be able to charge them making them ineffective. They are however useful during summer or in other circumstances when you are in isolation and need a power source.

Crank lights

These lights are good for an emergency if you don't have anything else. However, they take a lot of hand cranking to power the tiny internal generator and the charge doesn't last very long so I wouldn't recommend relying on these as your only lighting source (you will quickly become tired of having to crank them every few minutes!)

LED head lights

These small lights are a good investment and very handy as they let you keep your hands free. You'll need one for each member of your household. Again, check the batteries regularly to ensure they are working properly.

Candles

Candles are inexpensive and easy to purchase from your local supermarket. They are however a safety risk and should not be let unattended or within reach of children or pets.

Keep them away from curtains, long hair and other flammable materials.

Make sure the candle holder has a wide base, so the wax does not drip onto the surface below.
If using candles, be sure to have a fire extinguisher within your home in case of an accident.

Most candles do not give off a large amount of light. To help increase the light quality, place your candle in front of a mirror. The flame's reflection will increase the amount of light in the room. Larger width candles with thicker wicks will give more light than thin candles.

Battery operated candles are also available that operate on a sensor and light up when it becomes dark.

Oil lamps

Oil lamps are not as popular as they once were, primarily because of the odour which can give some people headaches and the safety risk.

Most hardware stores sell oil lamps, spare wicks and globes.

To increase their light, place the oil lamp in front of a mirror.

Never leave children or pets unattended with an oil lamp and make sure you have a fire extinguisher available in your home in case of accidents.

After each use, trim the wick and clean the globe. This will maximize light output and decrease smoke and soot.

How much water do you need?

This book is looking at what you need for a short-term lockdown. Most people do not have enough space within their homes to store water for a long-term situation. A water tank or other water source would be preferable for this type of scenario.

How much water do you need?

If you would like to store water at your home, you need to figure out how much water you and the members of your household including pets need for a minimum of three days.

Bottled water is one of the first items to disappear from supermarket shelves when a storm, pandemic or other natural disaster is heading your way, so it is a good idea to have what you need safety stored away.

The CDC (Centre of Disease Control) https://www.cdc.gov/ recommends each person needs 4 litres/1 gallon of water per day. This includes 2 litres/2 quarts for drinking and cooking and 2 Litres/2 quarts for washing up.

Storing tap water

Use heavy duty containers with a lid.

Do not use milk containers as these are usually made from PET (polyethylene terephthalate)

which is porous, difficult to clean and only made for short-term use. Because of its porous nature, bacteria and algae can grow inside the containers when not refrigerated.

Do not use containers that have held poisons or chemicals.

Larger barrels of water can be stored; however, smaller ones are preferable. If there is a leak or the water becomes contaminated, all your water won't be lost if you have it stored in several containers.

Method for cleaning
Wash your empty containers in hot soapy water, then rinse twice. Fill the container with water and 1 Teaspoon of bleach. Let sit for 10 minutes. Pour out water and fill with clean, room temperature tap water. Store in a dark cool place. The slight residue of bleach will help prevent bacterial growth.

How to freeze vegetables

Before freezing your vegetables, it is a good idea to cut them into smaller pieces and blanch them in boiling water for a few seconds. This kills any bacteria and slows vitamin and mineral loss.

After blanching your vegetables lay them on a sheet of baking paper to cool before placing in zip lock bags and freezing. You can then take whatever you need from the back and return the rest to the freezer.

To blanch
Fill a large pot with water and bring to the boil.
Add vegetables (about two cups of chopped vegetables depending upon the size of your pot), cover, return to a boil and cook. See suggested blanching time for vegetables below.
Transfer the vegetables to a large bowl of iced water. Drain well, pat dry.

Suggested Blanching times for vegetables

Asparagus
Prep: Trim woody ends.

Blanching Time: 2-3 minutes

To Reheat Frozen Vegetables (Microwave): 1-2 minutes

To Reheat Frozen Vegetables (Steaming): 2-3 minutes

Capsicum/Bell Peppers
Prep: Remove seeds; cut into pieces.

Blanching Time: 2-3 minutes

To Reheat Frozen Vegetables (Microwave): 1-2 minutes

To Reheat Frozen Vegetables (Steaming): 2-3 minutes

Broccoli & Cauliflower
Prep: Cut into florets.

Blanching Time: 3 minutes

To Reheat Frozen Vegetables (Microwave): 2-4 minutes

To Reheat Frozen Vegetables (Steaming): 2-4 minutes

Brussels Sprouts

Prep: Remove outer leaves, trim stems. Halve small sprouts or quarter larger.

Blanching Time: 2-3 minutes

To Reheat Frozen Vegetables (Microwave): 2-4 minutes

To Reheat Frozen Vegetables (Steaming): 4-6 minutes

Carrots

Prep: Peel and cut into slices or cubes.

Blanching Time: 2 minutes

To Reheat Frozen Vegetables (Microwave): 1-2 minutes

To Reheat Frozen Vegetables (Steaming): 2-3 minutes

Corn

Prep: Husk corn and use a knife to remove kernels.

Blanching Time: 2 minutes

To Reheat Frozen Vegetables (Microwave): 1-2 minutes

To Reheat Frozen Vegetables (Steaming): 2-3 minutes

Green Beans

Prep: Trim stem ends.

Blanching Time: 3 minutes

To Reheat Frozen Vegetables (Microwave): 1-2 minutes

To Reheat Frozen Vegetables (Steaming): 2-3 minutes

Freezing fruit

Fruit does not need to be blanched, only washed, however stones/pits should be removed, and fruit cut into pieces.

Blackberries, Blueberries & Raspberries

Prep: Wash and pat dry.

Blanching Time: N/A

Nectarines, Peaches & Plums

Prep: Remove pit; cut into sixths.

Blanching Time: N/A

Strawberries

Prep: Remove the stem and hull. Cut large ones in half.

Blanching Time: N/A

Lemons

Prep: Remove skin and quarter.

Blanching Time: N/A

Limes

Prep: Remove skins and quarter.

Blanching Time: N/A

How to sanitize your food

Fruits and vegetables

Wash fresh produce (fruits and vegetables) in warm soapy water to remove any contaminants, then rinse in fresh running water. Viruses can remain on surfaces for 3 days.

Fill sink with hot water and some detergent.
Fill a 2nd sink, bowl or bucket with cold water.
Separate leaves for lettuce etc. for easy access to clean.

Plunge fruit and vegetables into soapy water. Swish it around and scrub if necessary. Work in small batches to reduce time in water (they don't need to soak).

Wash under cold running water to rinse off soap.
Dry on a dish rack or similar to drain.
Store as you ordinarily do.

Meat, fish, seafood don't need to be sanitized as they are going to be cooked (usually over a high heat).

Food in cans, jars and packets usually don't need to be sanitized, however if you want to be extra cautious these can be stored separately from your other food for three days before adding to your pantry.

For vulnerable people (elderly and people with a low immunity)

For the elderly and people with a lower immunity, every item that enters the kitchen needs to be sanitized or separated for three days (e.g. in a box, separate fridge) before being put in the pantry/fridge.

This includes:

bottles and jars of sauces, spreads

cans of vegetables

packets of noodles, dried beans, frozen vegetables

bottles of fruit juice, drinks

packets/bottles of dried herbs

meat (wash the outside packaging)

Products in paper bags. These can be wiped with disinfectant wipes or sprayed and wiped.

toiletry products such as toothpaste, face wash, shaving cream and any other personal hygiene items, particularly those for the face, eyes and mouth.

Learn to cook in a crisis

What do you do if the power goes out? Do you have a back-up source for cooking? It could be a gas stove, BBQ, wood stove, portable camping stove or a portable Butane stove.

Gas stoves
If you have a gas stove, you will be able to use it in a power outage. You will, however, need a match to light the flame as the electrical ignition switch will not work.

BBQ

A gas BBQ or grill is a handy way to cook meat, fish and vegetables and many of the newer variety's come with a hood making it useful to cook a roast. If not connected to your house mains supply, you will need to keep a spare bottle of LPG gas available.

Wood stoves

Wood stoves with a flat top for cooking are a useful alternative. They can be used for heating and cooking and are free to use until your wood supply runs out.

They do however need to be installed profession-ally and have a chimney or flu to take smoke from the house outside. When cooking on a wood stove you will need cast iron cookware as this will withstand the higher temperatures of a woodstove. You can also cook inside the woodstove wrapping vegetables like potatoes in aluminum foil to slowly cook.

Camping Stove

A small portable stove is very useful in a power out-age or any situation where you cannot cook in your kitchen, for example during a flood where you need to move to higher ground. You will need either a gas bottle or butane gas cartridges to fuel the stove in-cluding a few spares. The stoves give off a good amount of heat and can be used to cook food and boil water from drinks. They are limited to only having one or two flames to cook on and you will need to cook in an area with good ventilation.

Sterno Stove

A Sterno stove relies on fuel made from gelled alco-hol and stored in a small can. They're portable and lightweight and can heat up tinned food quickly. You will need to have a good supply of the fuel cans on hand.

Solar Oven

A solar oven is another alternative to cooking; however, you will need ample sunlight for it to work. Foods with a high moisture content that can be cooked at a low temperature work best.

Before and during a storm

Food

If you have lost power or think you may lose power, move commonly used items such as milk, butter and eggs to an esky/cooler stocked with ice to keep them cold.

Keep other food in your refrigerator and freezer and keep the doors shut. Some foods in your freezer will thaw quicker than others and these should be consumed first such as ice cream and frozen berries.

Fill any empty spaces in your freezer with bags/containers of water as these will freeze and help to keep the other contents cold.

Place a sign on the refrigerator reminding household members not to open the door. Every time the door is opened, cold air flows out and warm air rushes in raising the temperature inside.

A full freezer will keep food frozen for 48 hours if left closed.

Cooking

Prepare your alternate cooking source (see chapter on cooking in an emergency) and extra fuel.

Lighting

Ensure you have candles, torches/flashlights etc. ready to use once the power goes out.

Emergency numbers

Have your list of neighbours, family and emergency numbers in an easily accessible spot to use if you need to.

First Aid

Keep a first aid kit and fire extinguisher close at hand in case of any accidents.

Generator

A fuel-based generator can be very useful during a storm. If your power goes out it can be used to power a small refrigerator and light for several hours depending upon the size.

After a Disaster

Food Supplies after a flood

Do not eat any food that has had any contact with floodwater as it can harbour dangerous pathogens. Dry food is particularly vulnerable as it is susceptible to mold and fungus.

Use gloves when handling any food that may have spoiled or be contaminated and wash your hands in warm soapy water.

If cans or jars of food are waterproof and undamaged, they can still be used. Remove the labels and wash the containers in hot, soapy water. Make a solution of 1 Tablespoon of bleach to 4.5 Litres/1 gallon and immerse the tins for 15 minutes. Remove tins and air dry for one hour before re labelling. Consume as usual, however, these should be used as soon as possible and not stored for a length of time. https://www.cdc.gov

Any cooking and eating utensils, plates, bowls etc. that have come into contact with flood water must also be sanitized.

After the power is restored

Check your food for safety.
If a power outage is less than 4 hours most of your food in your refrigerator should be fine as long as the door was kept closed. Perishable foods such as dairy products, lunch meats and seafood should be discarded.

Any thawed meat should be cooked immediately. If the power outage has been for an extended period or you are unsure, throw the meat away.

Check each package individually as smaller packets will thaw more quickly than larger ones. Food may look fine but harbour bacteria that can cause deadly food borne illnesses.

Easy Recipes for a lockdown

Chicken and vegetable Ramen noodles

Ingredients
- 2 packets of ramen or two-minute noodles. (other instant type noodles can also be used) Flavour sachet is not needed.
- 1 Tablespoon oil
- 2 garlic cloves crushed (garlic granules can also be used)
- ½ sliced onion
- 200g chicken thighs cut into small pieces (remove for a vegetarian version)
- 1 ¼ cups of water
- 1 small red capsicum/bell pepper (frozen can be used)

- 2 cups cabbage finely sliced
Sauce
- 1 Tablespoon soy sauce
- 1 Tablespoon Oyster sauce
- 2 teaspoons Hoisin sauce
- 1 Tablespoon Mirin

Instructions

Mix sauce ingredient together
Heat oil in a wok or frypan over high heat. Add onion and garlic and cook until starting to go golden. Be careful they don't burn.

Add chicken and cook until outside is white in colour.

Add sauce mixture and cook for one minute or until chicken is caramelized.

Add carrot and capsicum and cook for one minute.

Push the chicken and vegetable mixture to one side of the frypan and add water into the space.

Place dried noodles into the water, and simmer for one minute.

Toss noodle mixture through the vegetables and sauce until coated. Add chopped cabbage. Fold though for one minute and serve immediately.

Beef and Bean Enchiladas or Bean Enchiladas

Note: any frozen vegetables, beans, lentils or chicken mince can be added or substituted for beef the filling.

<u>Ingredients</u>

- 8 tortillas or burrito wraps
- 1.5 cups cheese (tasty, cheddar or mozzarella)

Enchilada Sauce
- 2 Tablespoons olive oil
- 3 Tablespoons flour
- 2 cups (500mls) chicken stock or vegetable if making vegetarian
- 1 ½ cups tomato passata
- Salt and pepper to season

Spice Mix
combine
- 1Teaspoon onion powder
- 1 Teaspoon garlic powder
- 1 Tablespoon cumin powder, paprika and dried oregano.

Filling
- 1 Tablespoon olive oil
- 2 garlic cloves crushed
- 1 brown onion finely chopped (dried onion flakes or frozen onion can also be used)
- 500g minced beef or 1 can refried beans
- 1 tin red kidney beans drained

Instructions

Make enchilada sauce
Heat oil in saucepan over medium heat, add flour and mix to a paste, cook for one minute, stirring continuously.
Add ½ cup chicken or vegetable stock and whisk until smooth. Slowly add remaining stock, passata, salt, pepper and two tablespoons of spice mix. Increase heat slightly, continue to stir until sauce thickens. Remove from stove.

Make filling

Preheat oven to 180C
Heat oil in frypan over high heat, add garlic and onion and cook for 2 minutes.
Add beef and cook for 2 minutes, add remaining spice mix and cook until browned. Add red kidney beans, salt and pepper and ¼ cup of enchilada sauce. Cook for 2 minutes then remove from heat.

Construct Enchiladas

Grease baking dish
Place filling in each tortilla, roll up then place in baking dish seam side down. Pour sauce over enchiladas and top with cheese. Bake in oven for 10-minutes covered with aluminum foil, then 10-minutes uncovered. Serve hot with a salad or vegetables.

One pot cauliflower, chicken and rice.

<u>Ingredients</u>

- 2 Tablespoons butter
- 1 Tablespoon olive oil
- 1 brown onion finely chopped (dried onion flakes or frozen onion can also be used)
- 2 garlic cloves crushed (garlic granules can also be used)
- 500g chicken thigh cut into small pieces
- 2 ½ Tablespoons of flour or cornflour
- 2 cups milk (fresh or long life)
- 2 cups of chicken stock (or use stock cubes in water)
- 1 ¼ cups white rice uncooked (long grain, jasmine or basmati)
- 1 teaspoon dried thyme (or other preferred herb)
- Salt and pepper
- ½ head cauliflower cut into florets (broccoli can also be used, or frozen vegetables thawed and drained of water)
- 2 cups grated cheese (mozzarella, tasty or cheddar)

Instructions

Melt butter and oil in a pot over high heat, add onion and garlic and cook for one minute. Add
chicken and cook until white in colour.
Turn heat down to medium, add flour and stir for
one minute. Slowly add milk to flour mixture, stir
continuously until thickened. Add stock, rice,
herbs, salt and pepper. Bring to a simmer then turn
down heat, cover and cook for twelve minutes
Add cauliflower and push into rice mixture until
covered. Cover again and cook for a further 3
minutes until cauliflower is just cooked.
Remove lid and stir through half the cheese. Top
with remaining cheese and grill. Serve hot.

Creamy chicken fettuccine

Ingredients

- 300g fettuccine or other dried pasta
- 2 Tablespoons butter
- 2 chicken breasts cut in half length ways
- Salt and pepper
- 2 garlic cloves crushed or garlic granules
- ½ cup dry white wine or extra chicken stock
- ½ cup chicken stock
- 1 ¼ cups thickened cream
- ¾ cup finely grated parmesan
- 70g baby spinach
- 100g sundried tomatoes if available

Instructions

Sprinkle chicken with salt and pepper on both sides. Melt butter in fry pan over high heat. Add chicken and cook for 2 minutes on each side until golden coloured. Remove chicken from pan, rest for a few minutes, then shred with 2 forks.
Cook pasta in large pot of salted boiling water. Drain pasta keeping one cup of the liquid to one side.

Make sauce by adding remaining butter and oil to frypan and melting over a medium heat. Add garlic

and cook until golden, add wine. Simmer rapidly stirring. Add chicken stock, cream, parmesan cheese and tomatoes. Simmer for 3-5 minutes string until sauce reduces and thickens.
Add pasta to sauce, tossing to coat. Add some of the reserved pasta liquid if the sauce is too thick. Serve hot with added grated parmesan if desired.

Creamy tuna pasta bake

Ingredients

- 350g penne pasta or other pasta
- 3 Tablespoons butter
- 3 garlic cloves crushed
- 4 Tablespoons flour
- 4 cups milk (long life milk can be used)
- 2 Teaspoons chicken or vegetable stock powder
- 1/2 cup parmesan cheese finely grated
- ½ Teaspoon of mustard powder
- ½ Teaspoon onion powder
- ½ Teaspoon garlic powder
- 425g canned tuna drained (salmon can also be used)
- 400g tinned corn drained (other tinned vegetables such as peas can be used)

Topping
- 1 ½ Tablespoons butter melted
- 1/2 cup panko breadcrumbs (other breadcrumbs may also be used)
- ¼ cup grated parmesan cheese
- ¼ Teaspoon salt

Instructions

Preheat oven to 180°C. Mix together topping ingredients and put to one side.

Cook pasta in a pot of salted boiling water until almost cooked then drain. Return to pot.

Make white sauce by melting butter in a large pot over medium heat, add garlic and cook until golden. Add flour and whisk. Gradually pour in milk. Add stock powder, mustard, onion and garlic powder. Turn down heat and cook until sauce thickens. Whisk continuously to ensure sauce does not burn. Remove from stove and stir in parmesan.

Add tuna into pasta and flake into large chunks with fork, add corn or other vegetable and pour over sauce stir through gently. Transfer mixture to a baking dish and top with crunchy topping. Bake for 25 minutes or until top is golden.

Chicken with Cashew nuts

Ingredients

- 500g chicken thigh/breast or tenders cut into small pieces or strips
- 2 Tablespoons peanut oil (vegetable oil can also be used)
- 2 garlic cloves crushed or garlic granules
- ½ onion chopped (white or brown)
- 1 green or red capsicum / bell pepper chopped into 2cm pieces
- 6 Tablespoons water
- ¾ cup roasted unsalted cashews

Sauce
- 1 Tablespoon corn flour/corn-starch
- 3 Teaspoons soy sauce
- 3 Tablespoons Chinese cooking wine or Mirin
- 3 Tablespoons oyster sauce
- 2 Teaspoons sesame oil

Instructions

Make sauce by mixing corn flour and soy sauce until there are no lumps. Add remaining sauce ingredients. Use tow tablespoons of the mixture to coat the chicken. Set aside for 10 minutes to marinate.

Heat oil over high heat in a wok or frypan, add garlic and onion and cook for one minute. Add chicken. Cook for two minutes then add the capsicum and cook for a further minute.
Next add the sauce mix and water. Bring to a simmer and cook until sauce thickens. Stir through cashews.

Serve with rice, cauliflower rice or Hokkien noodles.

Chilli con carne

<u>Ingredients</u>

- 1 Tablespoon olive oil
- 3 garlic cloves crushed (dried garlic can also be used)
- 1 onion diced (dried onion flakes or frozen onion can also be used)
- 1 red capsicum/ bell pepper diced (frozen can be used)
- 500g beef mince / ground beef
- 3 Tablespoons tomato paste
- 800g can crushed tomato
- 420g can red kidney beans drained (other beans can also be used)
- Pinch of salt

For a **vegetarian option** remove mince and add extra beans and tinned corn. Mince substitute and mushrooms can also be added.

<u>Spice mix</u>

    3 teaspoons of Mexican chilli powder **or**
- 1 Teaspoon cayenne pepper
- 1 Teaspoon paprika powder
- 1 Teaspoons cumin powder
- 1 Teaspoons garlic powder
- 1 Teaspoons onion powder

<u>To serve</u>
Rice or corn chips or baked potato
Grated cheese, sour cream

<u>Instructions</u>

Heat oil in a frypan over medium high heat. Add garlic and onion, cook for 1 minute. Add capsicum and cook until onion is translucent. Increase heat and add mince. Cook until brown.
Add spice mix, tomato paste and tinned tomato. Simmer stirring occasionally for 10 minutes.

Serve over rice, ladle into bowls and serve with corn chips, stir through pasta or use to stuff baked potatoes. The chilli can also be frozen for later use.

Curry cauliflower soup

Ingredients

- 1 cauliflower head cut into florets
- 200g potatoes peeled and chopped
- 1 brown onion sliced into rings
- 2 cloves garlic unpeeled (garlic granules may be used instead and added with other spices)
- 1 Teaspoon ground cumin
- 1 Teaspoon ground coriander
- 2 Teaspoons curry powder
- Salt and pepper
- ¼ cup olive oil
- 4 cups vegetable stock (or water)
- ½ cup milk (long life milk or substitute can be used)
- 1 ½ cups finely grated parmesan cheese

Instructions

Pre heat oven to 220C
Place cauliflower, garlic cloves with skin on, potato and onion on lined baking tray. Drizzle with olive oil. Roast for 25 minutes or until vegetables are tender.

Place vegetables and peeled garlic into a food processor with two cups of stock and blend until a smooth puree.
Transfer puree to a large pot, add remaining stock and milk. Add spices and bring to the boil. Stir in parmesan and season with salt and pepper.

Serve hot with crusty bread

Soup can be frozen for later use.

Baked Spaghetti

Ingredients

- 500g spaghetti
- 8 – 10 slices Swiss cheese or other cheese
- 2 cups (200g) mozzarella cheese grated

<u>Bolognese sauce</u>

- 2 Tablespoons olive oil
- 3 garlic cloves minced
- 1 onion chopped
- 1carrot finely diced (mix of tinned peas carrots and corn can also be used)
- 1 stick celery finely diced (optional)
- 750g beef mince/ground beef
- 3/4 cup (185ml) dry red wine (beef or vegetable stock may be substituted)
- Two tins crushed tomato
- ¼ cup tomato paste
- 2 Teaspoons Worcestershire sauce
- 3 dried bay leaves
- ½ Teaspoon oregano
- ½ teaspoon thyme
- ½ teaspoon garlic granules
- Salt and pepper

Vegetarian option remove mince and add red kidney beans or other tinned drained beans.

Instructions

Pre heat oven to 180C 350F
Heat oil in a frypan over medium high heat, add
garlic and onion and cook until translucent. Add
celery and carrot. Cook for 3 minutes.
Turn up heat, add mince and cook until brown.
Add wine (or stock) and spices and simmer for
two minutes. Add Worcester sauce, tomato paste
and tinned tomato and stir through. Simmer over
low heat for 20 minutes. Stirring occasionally so as
not to burn bottom. Add water if too much sauce
evaporates. Add salt and pepper.

While sauce is simmering, cook pasta in large pot
of salted boiling water for 10 minutes or until al
dente. Drain and return to pot. Add half the sauce
and stir through.
Spread half the pasta in a casserole dish, layer with
half remaining sauce. Top with cheese slices, then
remaining pasta and remaining Sauce. Finish with
grated mozzarella.
Cover loosely with foil and bake for 25 minutes.
Remove foil and bake for a further 10 minutes.
Cut slices with a knife and use a spatula to serve
pieces like a lasagna!

Can be frozen and reheated in microwave.

Chicken or Salmon Yakitori Skewers

Ingredients

500g chicken thigh fillets or salmon with skin removed
¼ cup Mirin
1/3 cup soy sauce
2 Tablespoon honey
2 Tablespoons sesame oil
2 Teaspoons ginger finely grated
1 clove garlic crushed
2 red onions chopped into squares
1 red capsicum cut into squares
Olive oil
Bamboo skewers (soak in cold water for 10-minutes before use to prevent burning)

Instructions

Whisk together mirin, soy sauce, honey, sesame oil, ginger and garlic in a jug. Place chicken or fish in a shallow dish, pour half the marinade mixture over the top, cover with plastic wrap and chill for 30 minutes.
Cut capsicum and red onions into squares. Drain chicken or fish. Thread chicken (or fish), capsicum and onion alternately onto skewers.

Cook skewers in a frypan with a little olive oil or under a grill or on the BBQ. Turn regularly, brushing with remaining marinade. Cook for approximately 10 minutes or until cooked.

Serve with rice, pasta or vegetables.

Shepard's Pie Parcels

<u>Ingredients</u>

- 1 Tablespoon olive oil
- 1 brown onion finely chopped (dried onion flakes or frozen onion can also be used)
- 1 carrot finely chopped
- 1/3 cup frozen peas
- 300g beef mince/ground beef
- 1 Teaspoon dried oregano
- 2 Tablespoons tomato paste
- 1 ½ Tablespoons Worcestershire sauce
- 1 Tablespoon flour
- 4 sheets of frozen, thawed puff pastry.
- ½ cup grated cheddar, tasty or mozzarella cheese
- 1 egg beaten
- 4 large potatoes peeled and chopped
- 2 Tablespoons milk
Tomato sauce to serve (optional)

Vegetarian version remove beef and use drained tinned beans, chopped mushrooms or meat alternative instead.

Instructions

Pre-heat oven to 220C, line two large baking trays with baking paper.
Heat oil in a large frypan over medium high heat.
Cook onion and carrot for 5 minutes stirring. Add mince and oregano, cook until browned.

Add tomato paste, sauce and flour stir for 30 seconds then add ½ cup water, bring to the boil. Stir in peas, cook for 2 minutes until sauce thickens.
Set aside to cool.
Cook potatoes in salted boiling water until soft, drain and add milk, mash until smooth.

Cut each pastry sheet in half to form 8 rectangles.
Place 4 rectangles on prepared trays. Place mince, potato and cheese on each rectangle. Top with remaining pastry. Using a fork, press edges of pastry together to seal.
Brush tops of pastry with beaten egg.
Bake in oven for 30minutes or until golden.

Serve with tomato sauce if desired, steamed vegetables or salad.

Vegetarian Bolognese

Ingredients

500g spaghetti or other pasta
2 Tablespoon olive oil
1 brown onion finely diced (onion flakes or frozen can also be used)
2 garlic crushed (garlic granules or powder can also be used)
1 carrot finely diced
1 celery stick finely diced
4 mushrooms chopped
1 red capsicum finely diced (frozen can also be used)
420g can lentils drained
½ cup water
1 Teaspoon oregano
Pinch salt

Instructions

Heat oil in a frypan and add onion and garlic, cook until translucent. Add carrot, celery, capsicum and mushroom, cook until tender. Stir in herbs, salt, tomato and half cup of water, bring to the boil. Reduce heat and simmer for 10 minutes. Stir in lentils and cook for 2 minutes

Cook spaghetti in salted boiling water until cooked.
Serve pasta topped with lentil Bolognese. Grated tasty or parmesan cheese can be sprinkled on top if desired.

This Bolognese sauce can also be used to stuff baked potatoes, just add sour cream and cheese on top and place in oven until potato is cooked.

One pot lemon chicken and rice

<u>Ingredients</u>

- 5 chicken thighs, skin on with bone
  <u>Marinade</u>
- 2 lemons
- 1 Tablespoon dried oregano
- 4 cloves garlic crushed (garlic granules can also be used)
- ½ teaspoon salt

<u>Rice</u>
- 1 ½ Tablespoons olive oil
- 1 small onion finely chopped
- 1 cup long grain rice
- 1 ½ cups chicken stock
- 1 Tablespoon dried oregano
- ½ teaspoon salt
- Pepper

<u>Instructions</u>

Combine chicken and marinade ingredients in a zip lock bag and leave for 30 minutes.
Pre heat oven to 180C

Remove chicken from marinade but, retain marinade
Heat ½ tablespoon of olive oil in a fry pan over medium high heat, cook chicken skin side down and cook until golden brown and turn and cook other side. Remove chicken and set aside.
Wipe oil from frypan using a paper towel. Heat 1 Tablespoon of olive oil in frypan and add onion and cook until translucent.

Add remaining rice ingredients and remaining marinade. Simmer for 1 minute then add chicken pieces on top of rice. Place lid on top of frypan or use aluminum foil. Bake in oven for 35 minutes. Remove lid and bake for another 10 minutes or until liquid is absorbed and rice is tender.
Remove from oven and rest for 5-10 minutes before serving. Garnish with zest of lemon and serve.

Mexican beef and rice casserole

Ingredients

- 2 Tablespoon olive oil
- 1 onion finely chopped (onion flakes or frozen can also be used)
- 3 garlic cloves crushed (garlic granules can also be used)
- 500g mince beef
- 1/3 cup tomato paste
- 1 ¼ cups white long grain rice
- 2 1/2 cups chicken stock (stock cube and water can also be used)
- 400g can corn kernels drained (frozen can also be used)
- 400g red kidney beans drained (other beans can also be used)
- 1 capsicum/bell pepper diced (frozen can also be used)
- 1 cup spring onion chopped
- 2 cups grated cheese

Mexican spices

- ½ teaspoon cayenne pepper (optional)
- 2 teaspoons dried oregano
- 3 teaspoons cumin
- 3 teaspoons coriander
- 3 teaspoons onion powder

- 2 teaspoons paprika
- ½ teaspoon salt

Vegetarian version remove meat and add extra beans, meat alternative or cooked vegetarian sausages sliced.

Instructions

Heat oil in large pot over high heat, add garlic and onion and cook unit translucent.
Add beef and cook until brown. Add Mexican spices and cook for one minute
Add tomato paste, stock, capsicum and rice. Stir and cook for one minute.

Add corn and beans, cover and simmer over medium for 15 minutes. Remove lid, stir through spring onion and half cheese.
Smooth top and sprinkle with remaining cheese.
Cover and leave for one minute for cheese to melt.

Serve

Can be frozen and reheated in microwave.

Apple Pikelets /flapjacks

Ingredients

2 cups self-rising flour
2 Tablespoons sugar
1 cup milk (long life milk can be used)
1 egg or powdered eggs
Canned apple
Cinnamon powder
1 Tablespoon butter or margarine

Instructions

Sift flour into a bowl. Add sugar, egg and milk and whisk until lump free. Add cinnamon and drained tinned apple and stir through.

Heat butter or margarine in a frypan over medium heat. Add Tablespoons of mixture to the frypan and cook until bubbling then flip pikelets and cook on other side. Serve hot or cold.

Flour Tortillas

Ingredients
2 cups flour
Pinch salt
1 teaspoon baking powder
¼ cup vegetable oil
½ cup warm water

Instructions
Mix together ingredients to from a dough. Cover with cling wrap or a dishcloth and let sit for 30 minutes in a warm spot.
Heat a frypan over medium heat. Divide dough into eight balls and roll each out into a circular shape on a floured board.
Fry in a dry pan until brown spots appear on the bottom. Flip the tortilla and cook on the other side until done.
While tortillas are hot fill with savoury filling such as beans, cheese and salsa. Or sweet such as honey and fruit.

Making bread by hand

If you don't own a bread machine, you can make your own bread by hand. It is easy to do and gives you a workout at the same time!

Ingredients

350ml lukewarm water
600g bread flour
2 teaspoon dried yeast

Instructions

Preheat oven to 220C
Place flour in a large mixing bowl. Add water and yeast and mix to form a dough.
Lightly flour your benchtop and knead the dough by hand vigorously until it is smooth and elastic. Knead for 12 minutes.

Return dough to mixing bowl and cover with cling wrap or a dishcloth making sure there is enough room for the dough to rise. Place in a warm spot for 40 minutes.

Remove dough from bowl and knead lightly on a floured surface for two minutes to de-gas the dough.
Place in an oiled bread/loaf tin and bake dough in oven for 30- minutes or until golden.

To test whether bread is cooked, tap lightly. Loaf is cooked when you hear a hollow sound.

Allow to cool for a few minutes before slicing.

Once cool, bread can be placed in a plastic bag or container to keep fresh.
Bread can also be frozen.

Make your own hand sanitizer

The best way to sanitize your hands is with soap and running water. Hand sanitizer is also a good way to sanitize, especially if you are away from home, however, hand sanitizer is usually one of the first items to become unavailable in stores during a public health crisis. You can make your own sanitizer, however, be sure to have at least 70% alcohol or the sanitizer will not be strong enough to kill bacteria and viruses. Do not use whiskey, vodka etc. as it is not strong enough.

Gel recipe

Ingredients
1/3 cup Glycerin or Aloe Vera Gel
2/3 cup 99% Rubbing Alcohol (isopropyl alcohol)
8-10 drops tee tree, lemon, peppermint or lavender essential oil (or your favourite)
Funnel
Pump or squeeze bottle/s
Jug for mixing

Instructions
Make sure you have clean hands before starting.
Sanitize bottles, jug and funnel by washing in hot water.
Mix together all ingredients and pour into bottles.
The World Health Organisation recommends you

let your concoction sit for 72 hours before using to ensure any bacterial introduced during the mixing process is killed.
https://www.who.int/gpsc/5may/Guide_to_Local_Production.pdf

Spray recipe

Ingredients

340 ml/12 oz Isopropyl alcohol
2 Tablespoons Glycerol or glycerin
1 Tablespoon Hydrogen peroxide
85 ml/3 oz Distilled water (or tap water boiled and cooled)
Mixing jug
Funnel
Spray bottles

Instructions

Sanitize jug, funnel and spray bottle by washing in hot water.

Mix together alcohol, glycerol (this helps to stop the alcohol from drying your hands out, however, you can make the mixture without it, just moisturize your hands afterwards), hydrogen peroxide and water. Por into spray bottles.
This mixture can also be used on a paper towel to use as a wipe.

Make an Oral Rehydration preparation

While children, the sick and elderly are most at risk of dehydration, anyone can suffer the effects of dehydration and it can even be fatal if severe enough and not treated. Most pharmacies have oral supplies of ready to use rehydration liquid or powder available, and a supply should be kept in your medical first aid kit at home. If you are not able to go to a pharmacy because you are in a lockdown/isolation situation, you can make your own oral rehydration preparation using goods you will have in your home.

Ingredients

4 Tablespoons lemon juice
½ cup honey
½ teaspoon salt
1 Litre/1000ml/ 1-quart warm water

Instructions

Mix all ingredients together and sip slowly to replenish the body's electrolyte balance.

Acknowledgments

Centre of Disease Control https://www.cdc.gov

World Health Organisation
https://www.who.int/gpsc/5may/Guide_to_Local_Production.pdf

| SILVERGUM PUBLISHING